Essential Oils and Aromatherapy Recipes

Essential Oils and Aromatherapy Recipes

Natural Health and Beauty Solutions Using Essential Oils and Aromatherapy for Stress Reduction, Pain Relief, Skin Care, and Beauty

Sheila Mathison

Softpress Publishing

SOFTPRESS PUBLISHING
4118 Hickory Crossroads Road
Kenly, NC 27542
softpresspub@gmail.com

ISBN-10: 1-4997-3039-x
ISBN-13: 978-1-4997-3039-5

Disclaimer:
The following statements have not been evaluated by the Food and Drug Administration. This product is not intended to diagnose, treat, cure, or prevent any disease. The advice and strategies contained herein may not be suitable for every situation. This work is sold with the understanding that the publisher is not engaged in rendering medical or other professional advice or services. The publisher does not specifically endorse any company or product mentioned or cited in this document. Websites listed were accurate at the time of publishing but may have changed or disappeared between when it was written and when it is read.

No responsibility or liability is assumed by the publisher for any injury, damage or financial loss sustained to persons or property from the use of this information, personal or otherwise, either directly or indirectly. While every effort has been made to ensure reliability and accuracy of the information within, all liability, negligence or otherwise, from any use, misuse or abuse of the operation of any methods, strategies, instructions or ideas contained in the material herein, is sole responsibility of the reader.

All information is generalized, presented for informational purposes only and presented "as is" without warranty or guarantee of any kind.

All trademarks and brands referred to in this book are for illustrative purposes only, are the property of their respective owners and not affiliated with this publication in any way.

Table of Contents

Introduction

Essential oils provide us with a natural way to enhance our lives and heal our ailments. They have been used for thousands of years to cure our physical ailments, boost our moods, and soothe our mental state. Essential oils were used long before modern medicines were even thought of and continue to be sought after to create relief from what ails us without all the undesirable and potentially harmful side effects contemporary pharmaceuticals can cause.

I have carefully crafted this handy reference so you will receive maximum benefit in your daily life from the many advantages offered by essential oils. This book is meant to be a useful guide to those who already have some familiarity with essential oils. Inside this valuable resource, you will find over **177 Recipes** for treating everything from sprains, to back pain, to headaches as well as useful, money-saving instructions for making your own toothpaste, lip balm, and hair care products, **plus tons more!**

Chapter 1 gets you started on the right foot with a complete list of tools and supplies you can use to make blending, storing, and using the oils safe and easy. I've even included a comprehensive index at the back to make it super simple and easy for you to find exactly the recipe you need in a hurry.

- Got a stuffy nose? See chapter 4.

- Need First Aid? See chapter 6.

- Want to make your own perfume or cologne? Chapter 7 has just the thing.

- Acne relief, sunscreen, preventing stretch marks, and even massage oils can be found in chapter 2.

Further, this book is a follow up to my first book, **Essential Oils and Aromatherapy Basics: Your Ultimate Guide to Getting Started and Safely Using Essential Oils to Beat Stress, Cure Your Ailments, Boost Your Mood, and Provide Emotional Wellbeing**. Please get this book for an indispensable primer on essential oils. It is packed with a wealth of useful information gathered from reliable and highly regarded sources. This comprehensive resource contains numerous helpful tips and guidance on buying, storing, and using essential oils so you can get started on the right path with confidence.

One last thing, as a way of saying Thank You for buying my book, I have put together a **FREE GIFT** just for you!

"25 Health and Beauty Recipes for Essential Oils"

This gift is the perfect complement to this book so just head over to this web address to get the free download:

https://tinyurl.com/yy5rhpp3

Chapter 1 - Tools and Supplies

There are some things you will need in order to get the most use out of your essential oils. As you probably already know, essential oils are very powerful and can actually be very corrosive. You will need to have some tools dedicated to mixing your essential oil blends. While essential oils are completely safe to use on your skin with a carrier oil, you cannot store your mixtures in plastic containers for most recipes. Mixtures like shampoos, lotions, and some soaps are safe to store in plastic containers as long as the essential oils are diluted. Pure oils in a single carrier oil should not be stored in plastic.

The following list will help you get started with your essential oil recipes:

- Glass dropper
- Double boiler (typically found in candle making or soap making supply sections)
- Glass bottles with stoppers—clear and amber-colored
- Glass spray bottles
- Silicone molds
- Small glass or metal containers
- Diffuser

- Roll-on vials
- Lip balm tubes
- Variety of carrier oils
- Beeswax
- Glass stirring rods
- Castile soap liquid and flakes
- Essential oils (take a look at the beginning of each chapter to discover the top 10 most common oils used in recipes within that chapter. You will find there are about 20 oils that are commonly used for recipes in each chapter.)

Many of these items you can use over and over. There will be an initial investment cost up front, but ultimately, you will save money by making your own natural products at home instead of buying them from the store. Don't be afraid to recycle jars from your pantry or refrigerator. Jelly jars, mayonnaise jars, and other jars can all be washed and used to hold your essential oil recipes.

The following links are some of the places you can buy your supplies online. Typically, it will be cheaper to buy in bulk from an online distributor than your local supply store. Check for coupons or other deals offered to new customers or percentages off for orders over a certain dollar amount.

http://www.wholesalesuppliesplus.com/Essential-Oils.aspx

https://www.aromatools.com

http://www.aromatics.com

http://www.bulkapothecary.com

TOOLS AND SUPPLIES

Don't forget to check Amazon for some really great deals on everything you need to get started. As always, check a seller's reputation before buying and be wary of buying essential oils from anybody that does not have an excellent reputation.

You can also buy shampoo and soap bases from most essential oil supply stores. All you need to do is add your essential oils, and the product is ready to use. This can save you some time and money by reducing some of the supplies you will need to buy up front.

Chapter 2 – Skin Care

Our skin is important to our overall health and self-esteem. Healthy, glowing skin looks great and makes you feel good all over. When your body is healthy on the inside, it will reflect on the outside. We put our skin through quite a bit in our daily routines. Sun damage, exposure to chemicals, and daily cleaning can leave our skin dry, cracked, and prone to rashes. You can help protect and heal your skin with a variety of essential oil treatments.

Massages are not just for luxury. They are therapeutic and when combined with essential oils, there are plenty of recipes that can be used to heal a variety of health conditions while leaving a person feeling better inside and out without ever having to swallow a pill.

Top 10 Essential Oils for Skin Care

- Lavender
- Cedarwood
- Tea tree
- Neroli
- Peppermint
- Rose

- Geranium
- Lemon
- Palmarosa
- Clary sage

You will notice carrier oils are mentioned throughout this book. As a point of reference, these are a few of the most common carrier oils and their typical uses:

- **Almond** - moisturizes, protects, and heals the skin
- **Coconut** - non-greasy, moisturizing oil that will leave skin smooth
- **Grapeseed** - very light, leaves a sheen when rubbed on the body
- **Jojoba** - easily absorbed by the skin, non-greasy, excellent for sensitive skin
- **Olive** - excellent moisturizer for hair, heavy oil
- **Rose hip** - ideal facial moisturizer, reduces appearance of flaws
- **Sunflower** - anti-inflammatory, protects and moisturizes the skin

Lotions

Making your own healing lotions is easy. You'll basically add several drops of essential oil to a carrier oil and apply it to the affected area. The following recipes tell you all you need to know to create your own lotions for wellness and beauty.

Eczema Relief

    1 tablespoon of coconut oil
    3 drops of lavender oil

Mix well and apply to skin. The coconut oil is light enough to apply during the day. You could use jojoba oil and lavender for night time. Lavender will help reduce itching.

Skin that is cracked from scratching could benefit from adding a drop of frankincense, geranium, myrrh or helichrysum oil. Those with eczema should always try one oil at a time to determine if there is an allergic reaction or increase in symptoms.

Eczema Cream

    ½ cup shea butter
    20 drops geranium oil
    30 drops cedarwood oil
    20 drops lavender oil

Mix ingredients together using a glass rod or metal spoon. Store in a glass jar with a lid. Apply to area once a day.

Anti-Wrinkle Formula

    10 drops neroli oil
    10 drops lavender oil
    10 drops frankincense oil
    10 drops rosemary oil
    10 drops fennel oil
    3 drops lemon oil
    10 drops carrot seed oil
    10 drops evening primrose oil

2 tablespoons sweet almond oil

Mix all ingredients in an amber-colored bottle. Apply to face and neck area every night before bed.

Moisturizing/Daily Use

½ cup coconut oil
5 drops of lavender essential oil
1 teaspoon of tea tree oil

Mix well in glass jar. Put a lid on the jar and use lotion once a day to help moisturize dry skin. This lotion can be used on the face, but do not get it near your eyes.

Sunscreen

Coconut is the best carrier oil to use for this purpose as it already has some natural SPF qualities. Add a few drops of eucalyptus oil (also natural SPF) and lavender oil. You will need to reapply your oil frequently for best results. This provides minimal protection from the sun, but it is completely safe. You will want to add 5 to 6 drops of an essential oil to every ounce of carrier oil. NEVER use a citrus oil in a sunscreen or other lotion if you are going to be in the sun.

Treating Sunburn - 1

Fractionated coconut oil or water
20 drops of lavender oil
2 drops of peppermint oil

Mix well and spray on the burned skin. Apply every 2 hours.

Treating Sunburn - 2

Aloe vera gel

4 drops lavender oil

Add lavender oil to 1 ounce of aloe vera gel and rub into skin for quick relief.

Heat Rash

½ cup baking soda
2 drops of lavender oil

Mix well and add to a tepid bath. For children over 10, you can add 4 drops of lavender.

Acne Relief - 1

Water
Tea tree oil

Mix 5 parts water to one part tea tree oil. Wash the acne prone area with the solution, being careful to avoid the eyes. Tea tree oil's antiseptic qualities are excellent for cleaning the pores. You can put the oil directly on the blemishes but test an area first.

Acne Relief - 2

Water
Lavender oil

Mix 5 parts water to 1 part lavender oil and use it as a toner for the skin. Use once a day or every other day depending on the skin's reaction to the remedy. For those who can tolerate the lavender without an adverse reaction, it is okay to dab some oil on a cotton ball and apply it directly to a pimple.

Athlete's Foot

5 drops tea tree oil

5 drops lavender oil
5 drops geranium oil
5 drops peppermint oil
5 drops myrrh oil
4 ounces coconut oil (or another carrier oil)

Mix well and apply to affected areas several times a day. The rash should be gone in a week, if not sooner.

Facial Mask - 1

Note: This is a good moisturizing mask
    2 tablespoons of almond oil
    2 tablespoons raw honey
    2 drops of either rose, lavender, or lemon essential oil

Massage onto skin and let sit for 15 minutes. Wash away with warm water.

Facial Mask - 2

For oily skin and those prone to acne, try this mask.
    2 teaspoons cosmetic clay (betonite clay is great)
    2 teaspoons nonfat yogurt
    2 drops lemongrass essential oil
    1 drop tea tree oil

Mix ingredients into a thick paste. Apply evenly to skin and let sit for 15 minutes. Wash away with warm water.

Facial Skin Toner

    8 ounces of distilled water
    2 drops lavender oil

1 drop palmarosa oil
1 drop rosewood oil

Mix ingredients in a bottle. Use a cotton ball to apply toner to face after each cleaning. Shake well before each use.

Preventing Stretch Marks

3 ounces cocoa butter
1 ounce avocado oil
4 drops neroli oil

Melt cocoa butter in a double boiler. Once melted, mix in avocado oil. Pour melted mixture into a small jar and allow to cool. Add the essential oil and mix well. Rub the butter mixture onto the upper thighs and stomach area to prevent stretch marks.

Massage Oils

There are various oils you will want to use depending on the situation and a person's mood. Mix ingredients and massage into the skin. Choose a carrier oil based on your preference. Light oils, like almond, are absorbed into the skin quickly while thicker oils like jojoba oil take longer and can feel a little heavy.

Anti-stress Oil

1 ounce carrier oil - almond is light and will absorb quickly
2 drops lemon oil
3 drops lavender oil
6 drops clary sage oil

Relaxing Oil

1 ounce carrier oil
10 drops Roman chamomile oil

Sore Muscles

1 ounce carrier oil
2 drops ginger oil
4 drops peppermint oil
5 drops eucalyptus oil

Aphrodisiac

1 ounce carrier oil
2 drops jasmine oil
8 drops sandalwood oil

Calming

1 ounce carrier oil
4 drops neroli oil
5 drops orange oil
6 drops petitgrain oil

Uplifting

1 ounce carrier oil
3 drops bergamot oil
3 drops eucalyptus oil
3 drops rosemary oil
3 drops lime oil
3 drops basil oil
5 drops spearmint oil

Invigorating

1 ounce of almond oil
4 drops peppermint oil
4 drops geranium oil
10 drops rosemary oil

You can mix the oils with a carrier oil for a massage or skip the carrier oil and add the blend to a warm bath.

Chapter 3 – Aches and Pains

It is virtually impossible to get through life without experiencing some aches and pain. Nearly every home in America has some kind of over-the-counter pain reliever stashed in a cupboard or a purse. These medicines usually contain warnings about what will happen if somebody takes too many within a certain amount of time and may even warn against common side effects like an upset stomach or vomiting. You may end up trading a headache for a stomach ache.

Essential oils can relieve your aches and pains quickly and safely. Experiment with some of the recipes below and make up a batch to keep on hand for the next time you strain a muscle or get a headache. You can create safe pain relievers that are quicker than anything you will ever find on a store shelf.

Top 10 Oils for Aches and Pains

- Peppermint
- Wintergreen
- Spearmint
- Lavender
- Chamomile
- Basil

- Oregano
- Marjoram
- Cedarwood
- Eucalyptus

Headaches - 1

2 drops of your carrier oil of choice
2 drops of peppermint, wintergreen, or spearmint oil

Mix together and apply to the back of your neck, temple area, under the nose, and your forehead.

Headaches - 2

8 drops lavender oil
4 drops Roman chamomile oil
1 ounce carrier oil

Mix together and apply to temples, back of neck, and forehead.

Headaches - 3

4 drops spearmint oil
4 drops eucalyptus oil
1 ounce carrier oil of your choice

Mix together and apply to temples, back of neck, and forehead.

Muscle Aches - 1

Mix 8 ounces (1 cup) of your chosen carrier oil with 16 drops of peppermint essential oil. You can use 28 drops of lavender oil instead of the peppermint if you prefer. Clary sage is another option, but you will only need 8 drops per 8 ounces of carrier oil.

Muscle Aches - 2

    1 tablespoon almond oil
    2 drops lavender oil
    2 drops cedarwood oil
    3 drops oregano oil
    4 drops peppermint oil

Mix together and rub into aching muscles.

Muscle Cramps - 1

Mix your chosen carrier oil with one of the following essential oils using a 1:1 ratio: juniper, basil, or marjoram are the best for relieving cramps or Charlie horses. Apply your mix to the affected area three times per day.

Muscle Cramps - 2

    1 ounce of almond oil or apricot oil
    3 drops pine needle oil
    4 drops lavender oil
    5 drops niaouli oil

Mix well and rub into affected area.

Sprains

    1 cup carrier oil
    4 drops cajuput oil
    8 drops eucalyptus oil
    10 drops marjoram oil
Mix well and apply to affected area three times a day.

Menstrual Cramps

    8 ounces of your chosen carrier oil

2 drops of basil, clary sage, or rosemary oil

Mix well and spread on stomach area. Place a warm towel over the area for 10 to 15 minutes.

Backaches

1 tablespoon almond oil
4 drops ginger oil
4 drops cardamom oil
4 drops wintergreen oil

Mix together and massage along spine and lower back area.

Strained Back

2 tablespoons coconut oil
10 drops lavender oil
6 drops rosemary oil
6 drops sandalwood oil
3 drops geranium oil

Mix all ingredients in a dark-colored jar. Massage oil on back before and after exercise.

General Pain

8 drops lavender oil
4 drops marjoram oil
1 drop cedarwood oil
1 drop chamomile oil
1 drop ginger essential oil
¼ cup carrier oil of your choice

Blend ingredients and store in a dark-colored jar with a lid. Apply to areas that ache.

Joint Pain

10 drops marjoram oil
8 drops eucalyptus oil
4 drops cajuput oil
2 drops black pepper oil
1 cup coconut oil

Mix all ingredients together. Rub on sore joints for pain relief.

Stomach Ache

1 teaspoon almond oil or coconut oil
1 drop of chamomile oil
1 drop clove oil
1 drop peppermint oil

Mix oils into your carrier oil of choice. Rub the mixture over the abdomen to help ease a stomach ache and cramping.

Chapter 4 - Illness and Allergies

The next time cold and flu season hits, reach for your essential oils instead of over-the-counter medicines that often cause a variety of unwanted side effects. Essential oils can provide relief from many of the symptoms that accompany various viruses, allergies, and other conditions without ever ingesting a single medicine. You will want to experiment with each of these recipes and adjust them to suit your individual needs and preferences.

Try a variety of carrier oils to determine which feels best on your skin. Some oils can be very heavy and take hours to absorb into the skin. If you are heading off to work, this may not be convenient. There is also a chance a person who is highly sensitive to smells may not be able to tolerate some of the stronger essential oils. There will be some trial and error as you figure out what works best for you and your family.

Important:
When mixing essential oils for children and babies, it is important to make sure the oils are diluted in a carrier oil. These recipes are designed for adults. It is advisable to cut the number of drops of essential oils in half when making a solution that will be used on a baby's skin.

Top 10 Oils for Illness and Allergies

- Eucalyptus
- Orange
- Lemon
- Peppermint
- Tea tree
- Lavender
- Rosemary
- Cinnamon
- Basil
- Thyme

Stuffy Nose - 1

Use a diffuser or boil a pot of water on the stove with eucalyptus oil. It helps clear the sinuses while disinfecting the air. It helps to lean directly over the boiling water and inhale the steam. Do this every hour or as needed.

Stuffy Nose - 2

2 ounces of jojoba oil
5 drops of peppermint oil
5 drops of tea tree oil
5 drops eucalyptus oil
20 drops lavender oil

Mix well. You can rub this around your sinus area, taking care to avoid your eyes. Make sure you rub a strip under your nose to help you breathe better. You can also diffuse this mixture into the air—minus the jojoba oil.

Vapor Rub

½ cup olive oil
2 tablespoons of beeswax pastilles
20 drops of eucalyptus oil
20 drops peppermint oil
10 drops rosemary oil
10 drops cinnamon oil

Use a double boiler to melt beeswax and olive oil together. Remove heat and add essential oils. Mix well and add to a jar with a lid. Allow to cool before using. Rub on chest and/or feet to help relieve congestion.

Cough

2 ounces of jojoba oil
5 drops cedarwood oil
5 drops eucalyptus oil
10 drops of lemon oil
10 drops of bergamot oil

Mix the oils together to create a chest rub. Rub the salve on your chest and back and the bottoms of your feet.

Allergy Symptoms (sneezing, watering eyes)

2 drops of laurel leaf oil
4 drops of eucalyptus oil
2 drops of fir oil
3 drops of Ravensara oil

Add oils to an inhaler or small amber-colored vial. When allergy symptoms arise, inhale the oil mixture.

Nausea

    4 drops of carrier oil

    2 drops of peppermint, ginger, nutmeg or patchouli oil

Mix well and dab a bit of the mixture behind each ear every hour until the nausea stops.

Vomiting

    1 drop basil oil

    1 drop peppermint oil

    1 drop lavender oil

    2 teaspoons of preferred carrier oil

Mix ingredients together. Rub the abdomen with the oil mix to stop the vomiting.

Sore Throat Rub

    4 drops chamomile oil

    1 drop thyme oil

    1 drop lemon oil

    1 drop tea tree oil

    1 teaspoon carrier oil

Mix oils together and rub mixture on neck area and behind the ears.

Sore Throat Steam Solution

    2 drops eucalyptus oil

    2 drops lavender oil

    1 drop thyme oil

Add the oil mix to the medicine cup of your vaporizer or add to a pot of boiling water on the stove.

Motion Sickness

   10 drops peppermint oil
   10 drops ginger oil
   10 drops chamomile oil

Mix the oils in a small jar with a lid. Inhale the combination to relieve the symptoms of motion sickness. You can put a couple of drops on a tissue and place it under the nose as well. It is best to do this before you get in the car or on a boat or train.

Rheumatism

   2 ounces carrier oil (jojoba is heavier and will be slowly absorbed by the skin. Alternatively, you can choose something light, like almond or coconut oil)
   6 drops juniper berry oil
   8 drops lavender oil
   10 drops rosemary oil

Mix well and apply as needed.

Bladder Infection

   8 drops juniper berry or cypress oil
   6 drops tea tree oil
   6 drops bergamot oil
   2 drops fennel oil
   3 tablespoons of a carrier oil

Mix ingredients together and rub oil onto abdomen and lower pelvic region once a day.

Arthritis Pain

   2 teaspoons of chosen carrier oil

4 drops of one of the following oils: cedarwood, eucalyptus, rose, geranium, frankincense, or peppermint oil.

Mix the oil into your chosen carrier oil and apply as needed. You can mix several of the oils together, but you will want to reduce the number of drops to make 4 total drops in the carrier oil.

Ear Infection

2 drops lemon oil
1 teaspoon coconut oil

Mix the lemon oil into the coconut oil. Rub the mixture just behind the ears and along the lymph nodes in the neck area.

Indigestion/Acid Reflux/Heartburn

2 drops eucalyptus oil
1 drop peppermint oil
2 drops fennel oil
1 teaspoon grapeseed oil

Mix ingredients together and rub on stomach area to relieve symptoms of indigestion.

Indigestion - 2

4 drops frankincense oil
1 teaspoon of chosen carrier oil

Mix together and rub over stomach area. This is very helpful to apply every night just before bed.

Menopause and/or Hot Flashes

10 drops clary sage oil

11 drops geranium oil

7 drops lemon oil

2 drops sage oil

2 tablespoons carrier oil

Blend oils together and use as a spot massage oil. You can skip the carrier oil and add the blend to a bath as well.

Menopause-Induced Night Sweats

10 drops grapefruit oil

10 drops lime oil

5 drops sage oil

5 drops thyme oil

2 tablespoons of carrier oil of your choice

Blend oils together and use as a spot massage oil. You can skip the carrier oil and add the blend to a bath as well.

ADHD

Vetiver oil

Add vetiver oil to a room diffuser. A study has proven when vetiver is diffused in a room, concentration of a child with ADHD improved by 100 percent. You can also add a few drops of vetiver oil to a tablespoon of a carrier oil and rub on the child's feet before sending off to school.

Autism

There are several oils that can be used to treat some of the symptoms associated with autism. Oils can be diffused into the room or mixed with a carrier oil and rubbed on a child's feet.

Vetiver - relaxes an over-stimulated mind
Cedarwood - calming
Lavender - calms the nervous system

Warts

12 drops lemon oil
4 drops tea tree oil
4 drops bergamot oil
4 drops thyme oil
4 drops cypress oil
1 tablespoon jojoba oil

Mix oils together and store in a jar. Apply the mixture once a day to the wart. For your children, increase the carrier oil to 2 tablespoons.

Ringworm

1 drop lavender oil
2 drops tea tree oil
1 teaspoon coconut oil
Add essential oils to coconut oil or other carrier oil and mix well. Apply to affected area with a cotton ball.

Varicose Veins

½ cup shea butter
¼ cup coconut oil
¼ cup jojoba oil
1 tablespoon vitamin E liquid
10 drops cypress oil
10 drops lemon oil
5 drops fennel oil
5 drops helichrysum oil

Mix shea butter and coconut oil in a double boiler and heat until mixture is melted. Remove from heat and add the oils and vitamin E. Refrigerate for 2 hours. Use an egg beater to whip the mixture into a heavy cream. Store mixture in a jar with a lid. Massage body butter onto legs and arms to promote circulation. Body butter is good for about six months.

Mouth Sores

6 drops myrrh oil
10 drops tea tree oil
1 drop peppermint oil
3 drops lemon oil
1 teaspoon almond oil

Mix ingredients together and store in a glass jar. Rinse mouth with about ½ ounce of the mixture once a day to relieve sores on the gums and inside the mouth. Do not ingest.

Corns and Callus Softener

12 drops lavender oil
6 drops myrrh oil
2 ounces sweet almond oil

Mix ingredients and store in a jar with a lid. Apply oil to calluses once a day to help soften.

Fibromyalgia

5 drops eucalyptus oil
1 cup hot water
1 compress pad or folded washcloth

Heat the water and add the eucalyptus oil. Dip the cloth in the mixture. Wring out the cloth and apply to sore area.

Fibromyalgia Massage Oil

4 drops eucalyptus oil
4 drops of rosemary oil
1 ounce sweet almond oil

Add the rosemary and eucalyptus oil to the carrier oil. Massage into area where there is muscle pain.

Constipation

15 drops rosemary oil
10 drops lemon oil
5 drops peppermint oil
2 tablespoons almond oil

Mix ingredients in a jar. Rub on abdomen three times a day.

Diverticulosis

3 drops rosemary oil
2 drops peppermint oil
1 drop chamomile oil
1 drop clove oil
1 teaspoon olive oil

Mix essential oils into carrier oil and rub over abdomen twice a day.

Shingles

10 drops sandalwood oil
5 drops blue cypress oil
4 drops peppermint oil

2 drops Ravensara oil
1 tablespoon carrier oil

Mix oils together. Rub mixture on affected areas one to three times a day.

Diuretic (for fluid retention)

4 drops of frankincense oil
5 drops of grapefruit oil
3 drops of laurel leaf oil
3 drops of lemon oil
5 drops of juniper berry oil
5 drops of cypress oil
2 ounces of a carrier oil

Mix essential oils in carrier oil. Store in a container with a lid. Rub on affected area five to six times a day.

Chapter 5 - Mental Health

Our daily lives are full of stress that can wreak havoc on our state of mind. It is not uncommon to feel sad, tired, anxious, or irritated after a long day at work. You may be unable to get a good night's rest, which only exacerbates the symptoms. Doctors will jump to prescribe anti-anxiety medicines and sleeping medicines to help improve your overall mental health. However, many of these prescription and over-the-counter medicines cause unwanted side effects that can make daily routines even more difficult.

Essential oils are an excellent way to balance your mood without worrying about suffering the consequences of a side effect. The oils can be used in a room diffuser or applied topically to the skin. You will want to keep a diffuser in the office and at home to help you manage stress, relax, or stay invigorated.

There are about 20 essential oils that are regularly used to balance the mood whether it is to calm a person's nerves or fight fatigue. You can opt to use a single oil or create a blend with complimentary oils. There are also plenty of companies who manufacture essential oil blends designed specifically for treating various moods. In many cases, it is quicker and more convenient to buy a blend already made than to buy several different oils to mix at home. At the end of the chapter, we will list blends that are available.

Top 10 Oils Used to Balance Mood

- Bergamot
- Orange
- Frankincense
- Jasmine
- Lavender
- Grapefruit
- Chamomile
- Ylang-ylang
- Vetiver
- Peppermint

You can make a large batch of the following 4 stress reducing recipes simply by multiplying by 5. Use these recipes in a diffuser or add a few drops to a warm bath.

Stress Reduction - 1

3 drops bergamot oil
1 drop geranium oil
1 drop frankincense oil

Stress Reduction - 2

3 drops clary sage oil
1 drop lemon oil
1 drop lavender oil

Stress Reduction - 3

3 drops grapefruit oil
1 drop jasmine oil
1 drop ylang-ylang oil

Stress Reduction - 4

2 drops Roman chamomile oil
2 drops lavender oil
1 drop vetiver oil

Anxiety Relief

1 teaspoon coarse sea salt
10 drops bergamot oil
4 drops lavender oil
4 drops orange oil
1 drop rose geranium oil
1 drop chamomile oil

Add the salt to a dark-colored bottle. Add the essential oils. You can keep this bottle in your purse or your drawer at work. When feeling tense or anxious, take off the lid and inhale three long breaths. You will instantly start to feel more relaxed.

The next four recipes for depression relief can be increased to use in a diffuser or added to a tablespoon of sea salt to carry around in a glass jar.

Depression Relief - 1

3 drops bergamot oil
2 drops clary sage oil

Depression Relief - 2

1 drop lavender oil
1 drop ylang-ylang oil

3 drops grapefruit oil

Depression Relief - 3

2 drops frankincense oil
1 drop lemon oil
1 drops jasmine oil

Depression Relief - 4

1 drop rose oil
3 drops sandalwood oil
1 drop orange oil

Depression Caused by Grief

10 drops rose absolute oil
4 drops sandalwood oil
4 drops neroli OR petitgrain oil
1 teaspoon sea salt

Mix all ingredients into small, dark jar with a lid. Inhale mixture from time to time when depression is bringing you down.

Anxious Depression

8 drops lavender oil
8 drops grapefruit oil
2 drops marjoram oil
1 drop chamomile oil
1 drop geranium oil
1 teaspoon coarse sea salt

Mix all ingredients in small, dark glass bottle. Smell the aroma from time to time to fight off depression.

Fighting Fatigue

Use an oil diffuser with peppermint oil. It gives you a natural energy boost. You can put a drop of peppermint oil (mixed with a carrier oil) on the back of the neck as well.

Mood Booster - 1

3 drops peppermint oil
3 drops lemon oil
3 drops orange oil

Mix together in a diffuser with the recommended amount of water for your device.

Mood Booster - 2

1½ ounces of water
20 drops sweet orange oil
20 drops bergamot oil
20 drops neroli oil
10 drops lavender oil
10 drops rose otto oil
10 drops frankincense oil
10 drops clary sage oil

Add water to a 2-ounce spray bottle. Drop in essential oils and shake well to mix. Spray your face (with eyes closed) for a quick mood enhancer.

Curbing Cravings

40 drops mandarin oil
20 drops lemon oil
12 drops peppermint oil
12 drops ginger oil

Add oils to a diffuser to help stop cravings for cigarettes, food, etc.

Relaxation Blend

    2 drops chamomile oil
    3 drops vetiver oil
    3 drops sandalwood oil

Pour in diffuser with manufacturer's recommended amount of water.

Harmonizing Blend

    2 drops cinnamon oil
    2 drops white fir oil
    3 drops patchouli oil

Pour in diffuser with manufacturer's recommended amount of water.

Insomnia - 1

Fill a bath with warm water and add 5 drops each of lavender and marjoram oil.

Insomnia - 2

Fill a bath with warm water and add 4 drops of chamomile and 2 drops of lavender oil.

Insomnia - 3

Add lavender or chamomile essential oil to a diffuser. Put the diffuser in your bedroom and let it run throughout the night.

You can add a couple of drops of one of these oils to your pillowcase as well.

Insomnia Blend

    1 ounce of coconut oil
    1 drop marjoram oil
    1 drop clary sage oil
    1 drop ylang-ylang oil
    2 drops Roman chamomile oil
    3 drops lavender oil

Mix oils together and massage into skin before bed.

Irritability Relief

    1 tablespoon coarse sea salt
    10 drops bergamot oil
    5 drops grapefruit oil
    4 drops sweet orange oil
    1 drop geranium oil
    1 drop ylang-ylang oil

Add sea salt to small, dark glass container. Add essential oils and mix well. This can be carried in your purse or stored in a desk drawer as a quick pick-me-up. Simply remove the lid and inhale the blend to find quick relief from crankiness.

Panic Attack Treatment - 1

    2 drops helichrysum oil
    3 drops frankincense oil

Put oils in diffuser or mix with 1 teaspoon of a carrier oil. You can also make a large batch and carry in a vial. When panic sets in, inhale the oils to settle your nerves.

Panic Attack Treatment - 2

1 drop rose oil
4 drops lavender oil

Put oils in diffuser or mix in with 1 teaspoon of a carrier oil. You can also make a large batch and carry in a vial. When panic sets in, inhale the oils to settle your nerves.

Anxiety Attack - 1

1 drops rose oil
4 drops frankincense oil

Put oils in a diffuser or mix in with 1 teaspoon of a carrier oil. You can also make a large batch and carry in a vial. When you start to feel anxious, inhale the oils to settle your nerves.

Anxiety Attack - 2

1 drop neroli oil
4 drops lavender oil
Put oils in a diffuser or mix in with 1 teaspoon of a carrier oil. You can also make a large batch and carry in a vial. When you start to feel anxious, inhale the oils to settle your nerves.

Feeling Lonely/Loneliness

1 drop rose oil
2 drops frankincense oil
2 drops bergamot oil

Put oils in a diffuser or mix in with 1 teaspoon of a carrier oil. You can also make a large batch and carry in a vial. When you start to feel the blues or alone, inhale the oils to give yourself a little pick-me-up.

Fighting Fear

    3 drops sandalwood oil
    2 drops orange oil

Put oils in a diffuser or mix in with 1 teaspoon of a carrier oil. You can also make a large batch and carry in a vial. To combat feelings of fear and anxiety, inhale the oils to calm your nerves.

Reducing Feelings of Anger/Frustration

    3 drops bergamot oil
    1 drop ylang-ylang oil
    1 drop jasmine oil

Put oils in a diffuser or mix in with 1 teaspoon of a carrier oil. You can also make a large batch and carry in a vial. To calm down and reduce feelings of anger, inhale the oils as often as needed.

Memory Booster

    4 drops cypress oil
    1 drop peppermint oil

Double or triple this recipe, if desired, to make into an inhaler solution. Use the oils alone in a diffuser or add to 1 tablespoon of a carrier oil to rub onto the skin.

Concentration Aid

    2 drops peppermint oil
    3 drops lemon oil

Double or triple this recipe if desired to make into an inhaler solution. Use the oils alone in a diffuser or add to 1 tablespoon of a carrier oil to rub onto the skin.

Oil Blends Available by Manufacturers

<u>Young Living</u> (https://www.youngliving.com)

    Peace and Calming Blend

    Present Time

    Citrus Fresh (calming blend)

<u>DoTerra</u> (https://www.doterra.com)

    Balance

    Elevation

    Serenity

    Citrus Bliss

Chapter 6 – First Aid

Life's little emergencies tend to have us reaching for our first aid kits or running for the nearest urgent care facility. Sometimes, it simply isn't possible or affordable to visit a doctor for minor problems. You can take care of many minor emergencies at home with your own first aid kit comprised of essential oils.

It is a good idea to keep some tonics and salves on hand that have already been pre-mixed. This insures the first aid medicines are readily accessible and you won't have to suffer in pain while you mix up a quick fix.

One of the benefits to essential oil treatments is the speed in which they work. You can find almost instant relief from pain when you opt to use essential oils. Some treatments may take a few minutes, but in general, essential oils work faster than any over-the-counter medicine you will find in your medicine cabinet.

Please note, young children have very sensitive skin, so you will want to use these remedies with caution. It is advisable to dilute the remedies to accommodate a child's sensitive skin. Always test an area first before rubbing any salve or lotion containing essential oils on a baby's skin.

Top 10 Oils for First Aid

- Peppermint
- Clove
- Tea tree
- Lavender
- Eucalyptus
- Chamomile
- Lemon
- Rosemary
- Cinnamon
- Clary sage

<u>Toothache - 1</u>

    3 drops clove oil
    ½ teaspoon olive oil

Mix oils together in a small bowl. Dip a cotton ball into the mixture. Place the cotton ball on aching tooth.

<u>Toothache - 2</u>

    1 tablespoon sunflower oil (carrier oil)
    6 drops tea tree oil
    4 drops Roman chamomile oil
    2 drops myrrh oil
    2 drops peppermint oil

Mix ingredients in a small jar. Apply to affected tooth as needed.

<u>Earache</u>

2 drops lavender oil
2 drops tea tree oil

Mix oils together. Dip a cotton ball in the mixture and place in each ear. Replace cotton ball two to three times a day. Do not put the oils directly into the ear.

Heat Exhaustion

Fill a bath with tepid water and add 6 to 8 drops of eucalyptus oil to help reduce body temperature.

Cuts - 1

Apply a few drops of tea tree essential oil directly to a cut. It has antibacterial qualities that will help disinfect a wound while promoting healing.

Cuts - 2

6 drops lavender oil
1 ounce witch hazel

Add witch hazel to bottle and drop in lavender oil. You can double or triple this recipe for a quick treatment for cuts and scrapes.

Cuts and Scrapes

This recipe is designed for you to make a jar of the mixture to add to your home's first aid supply.

3 ounces almond oil
1 ounce grated beeswax
40 drops lavender oil
40 drops tea tree oil

Use a double boiler to melt beeswax. Warm up your carrier oil and pour it into a bowl. Add the melted beeswax to the heated carrier oil and mix well. Add the essential oils and mix again. Pour the mixture into a glass jar and allow it to cool. Seal the jar with a lid. When you need a gentle ointment for a cut or scrape, clean the wound and add this mixture.

Asthma Attack

Asthmatics should not inhale essential oils. It is best to use a topical application rubbed onto the feet. Mix a carrier oil and 5 drops of peppermint, eucalyptus, rose, or frankincense essential oil. Rub the mixture onto the feet. You can also create a chest rub with a carrier oil and 5 drops of lavender oil. The lavender reduces the spasms that accompany a bout of asthma.

Fever

Fill a bowl with ice water. Add 1 drop of peppermint oil and 3 drops of lavender and stir the water, making sure the oils are thoroughly mixed in. Dip a washcloth into the water, wring out and place on the forehead. Repeat this until the fever has come down or the water is gone.

Burn Salve

   ¼ cup raw honey
   ¼ teaspoon lavender oil (Use only $1/8$ teaspoon of oil for
      babies and toddlers)

Mix oil and honey together and store in a jar with a lid. To treat a minor burn, run cold water over the area. Rub the salve over a burn as needed.

Bee Stings

   2 drops lavender oil
   1 drop wintergreen oil

1 drop chamomile oil

Make sure to remove stinger first! Mix oils together and apply 1 to 2 drops directly to sting area. Repeat every 15 minutes until the pain stops.

Hives
4 drops peppermint oil for cooling or lavender for soothing
1 teaspoon coconut oil

Mix coconut oil and either lavender or peppermint oil and dab directly onto the affected area.

Poison Ivy - 1
2 tablespoons water
2 tablespoons apple cider vinegar
1 teaspoon kosher salt
3 drops lavender oil
3 drops tea tree oil
3 drops peppermint oil

Mix all ingredients together in a glass jar. Apply mixture to affected area as needed. Store the jar in the refrigerator.

Poison Ivy - 2
4 ounces aloe vera gel
10 drops lavender oil
10 drops cypress oil
10 drops Roman chamomile oil

Mix all ingredients and apply as needed. This mixture will help stop the itching that accompanies a healing rash.

Scabies

2 drops cinnamon oil
2 drops rosemary oil
2 drops pine oil
1 drop thyme oil
1 teaspoon of carrier oil

Mix all ingredients and apply to affected areas.

Bruises

1 ounce jojoba or almond oil
8 drops helichrysum oil

Mix oils together and store in a dark-colored glass bottle. Rub oil on bruised areas for relief from the pain associated with bruising as well as the discoloration caused by a bruise.

Mosquito Bites

1 teaspoon coconut oil
5 drops lavender oil
1 drop peppermint oil

Mix oils and rub on bites for itch relief.

Fire Ant Bites

Cajeput oil

Apply oil directly to bites several times on the first day of the bites. You can switch to lavender oil in a carrier oil after the first day to help the skin heal.

Reduce Blood Pressure

10 drops lemon oil
10 drops sweet marjoram oil
10 drops ylang-ylang oil

30 drops clary sage oil

2 tablespoons almond oil

Mix ingredients in bottle. Rub on skin to reduce high blood pressure.

Antibacterial Tonic (Thieves Oil)

40 drops of clove oil

35 drops of lemon oil

20 drops of cinnamon oil

15 drops of eucalyptus oil

10 drops of rosemary oil

Mix oils together and store in an amber-colored jar with a lid. This recipe will make approximately 5 ml or a small bottle of Thieves Oil. To use Thieves Oil, you need to dilute it in water or a carrier oil before applying to wounds.

1 drop of Thieves to 4 drops of carrier oil,

OR

1 drop of Thieves to 1 ounce of water to create an antibacterial spray.

Chapter 7 – Perfumes and Colognes

Smelling good makes us feel good, but sometimes, perfumes and colognes that are made with synthetic ingredients are extremely harsh on our skin. They tend to be made with synthetic chemicals which further dries out the skin and causes even more problems. Cost is also an issue. It can cost a small fortune to smell good with some of the high-end fragrances sold in department stores.

You can create your own custom fragrance to suit your body and your preference with essential oil blends. These are a lot of fun to make and are excellent gifts for friends and family members. The following recipes are a starting point for you. At the end of the chapter, you will find a list of essential oils that are regularly used to create perfumes. You can certainly create your own blend by experimenting. Please note that essential oils tend to have much stronger aromas than perfumes you would buy in the store. A little goes a long way.

Body Spray
    8 ounces distilled water
    1 tablespoon witch hazel
    20 to 30 drops of your favorite essential oil

Pour your ingredients in a container and mix well. Make sure you shake well before spraying on your body. You can combine oils to create a signature scent.

Perfume - 1

    5 drops coriander oil
    6 drops bergamot oil
    4 drops neroli oil
    1 drops jasmine oil
    3 drops rose oil
    2 teaspoons jojoba oil

Put the jojoba oil in your container and add the essential oils in the order listed. Mix well and allow the mixture to sit for one week with the lid on.

Perfume - 2

    1 tablespoon jojoba oil
    1 tablespoon vodka
    8 drops sandalwood oil
    3 drops lavender oil
    1 drop cedarwood oil

Pour the jojoba oil and vodka in a dark-colored glass bottle. Add the essential oils and shake well. Allow the mixture to sit for 2 weeks before using to give the oils time to cure. Shake before each use. Store in a cool, dark place.

Perfume - 3 (Solid)

    4 tablespoons grated beeswax
    4 tablespoons jojoba, almond, or a mildly scented olive oil

30 drops sandalwood oil

30 drops vanilla oil (this will be sold in another diluted oil)

25 drops grapefruit oil

20 drops bergamot oil

Using a double boiler, melt beeswax until liquified. Add jojoba and remove from heat after the oil has mixed with the beeswax. Let the mixture cool to a "warm" level before adding the essential oils. Pour the mixture into metal containers or silicone molds. To use, dab your finger in the mixture and rub behind your ears, inside wrists, and along your neck.

Floral Perfume

1 tablespoon jojoba oil

1 tablespoon vodka

5 drops palmarosa oil

3 drops rose oil

1 drop rose geranium oil

1 drop ylang-ylang oil

Pour the jojoba oil and vodka in a dark-colored glass bottle. Add the essential oils and shake well. Allow the mixture to sit for 2 weeks before using to give the oils time to cure. Shake before each use. Store in a cool, dark place.

Lavender Perfume

1 tablespoon jojoba oil

1 tablespoon vodka

6 drops lavender oil

4 drops frankincense oil

1 drop rose geranium oil

Pour the jojoba oil and vodka in a dark-colored glass bottle. Add the essential oils and shake well. Allow the mixture to sit for 2 weeks before using to give the oils time to cure. Shake well before each use. Store in a cool, dark place.

Spicy Perfume

  1 tablespoon jojoba oil
  1 tablespoon vodka
  8 drops sandalwood oil
  2 drops orange oil
  1 drop patchouli oil
  1 drop ylang-ylang oil

Pour the jojoba oil and vodka in a dark-colored glass bottle. Add the essential oils and shake well. Allow the mixture to sit for 2 weeks before using to give the oils time to cure. Shake well before each use. Store in a cool, dark place.

Uplifting Perfume

  1 tablespoon jojoba oil
  1 tablespoon vodka
  5 drops bergamot oil
  5 drops grapefruit oil
  1 drop rose geranium oil

Pour the jojoba oil and vodka in a dark-colored glass bottle. Add the essential oils and shake well. Allow the mixture to sit for 2 weeks before using to give the oils time to cure. Shake before each use. Store in a cool, dark place.

Sweet-Smelling Perfume

1 tablespoon jojoba oil
1 tablespoon vodka
5 drops vanilla oil
4 drops cocoa absolute
1 drop ylang-ylang

Pour the jojoba oil and vodka in a dark-colored glass bottle. Add the essential oils and shake well. Allow the mixture to sit for 2 weeks before using to give the oils time to cure. Shake before each use. Store in a cool, dark place.

Youthful Perfume

1 tablespoon jojoba oil
1 tablespoon vodka
9 drops grapefruit oil
1 drop rose geranium oil
1 drop ylang-ylang oil

Pour the jojoba oil and vodka in a dark-colored glass bottle. Add the essential oils and shake well. Allow the mixture to sit for 2 weeks before using to give the oils time to cure. Shake before each use. Store in a cool, dark place.

Jasmine Perfume

1 tablespoon jojoba oil
2 drops jasmine oil
4 drops sandalwood oil
2 drops ylang-ylang oil

Mix ingredients in a dark-colored bottle. Allow perfume to cure for 24 hours before using. Apply as desired.

Men's Cologne

10 drops lavender oil
20 drops coriander oil
22 drops sandalwood oil
23 drops cedarwood oil
5 drop frankincense oil
7 tablespoons alcohol (vodka)

Pour the alcohol into a jar. Add the essential oils in order and mix well. Allow the mixture to sit for one week in order for the oils and scents to blend.

Men's Earthy Cologne

10 drops clove oil
20 drops white fir oil
40 drops bergamot oil
5 drops lemon oil
1 tablespoon coconut oil

Pour coconut oil into a roll-on liquid dispenser. Add essential oils and let the mixture sit for 24 hours. Rub cologne on as desired.

Spicy-Scented Cologne

36 drops cinnamon oil
12 drops cassia oil
12 drops peppermint oil
12 drops grapefruit oil
1 tablespoon coconut oil

Pour coconut oil into a roll-on liquid dispenser. Add essential oils and let the mixture sit for 24 hours. Rub cologne on as desired.

Woodsy-Scented Cologne

8 drops fennel oil
8 drops cypress oil
8 drops wild orange oil
32 drops sandalwood oil
8 drops lime oil
8 drops wintergreen oil
1 tablespoon coconut oil

Pour coconut oil into a roll-on liquid dispenser. Add essential oils and let the mixture sit for 24 hours. Rub cologne on as desired.

Musky Cinnamon Cologne

28 drops cinnamon oil
12 drops Rosemary oil
12 drops wild orange oil
1 tablespoon coconut oil

Pour coconut oil into a roll-on liquid dispenser. Add essential oils and let the mixture sit for 24 hours. Rub cologne on as desired.

Sweet Musk Cologne

32 drops lime oil
24 drops fennel oil
16 drops patchouli oil
1 tablespoon coconut oil

Pour coconut oil into a roll-on liquid dispenser. Add essential oils and let the mixture sit for 24 hours. Rub cologne on as desired.

Creating Your Own Signature Scent

Creating your own scent will take a lot of trial and error as you figure out which oils blend well for your particular tastes. Perfumes and colognes are typically made with a minimum of three different oils. These are referred to as notes.

Top Notes - This is typically the strongest scent you will add to your perfume. A top note is the scent you smell immediately after you apply the perfume. It is quick and powerful and disappears almost as quickly as it appeared. Your top note will last about 30 minutes.

Middle Notes - Middle notes start to appear about an hour after a perfume has been applied. The scent slowly builds and compliments the top note.

Base Notes - This is the essential oil that will last the longest when applied. It is more subtle and tends to be heavier than the top and middle notes.

When creating your own perfume, the ratio for top, middle, and base notes is as follows:

- Top notes - 3 drops
- Middle notes - 2 drops
- Base notes - 1 drop

When making your own perfume or cologne, you have the option of using different bases. If you prefer light and airy, alcohol bases are ideal. If you prefer not to use alcohol, you can opt for a carrier oil. The following are base recipes you can use to start your own perfume.

Please note, perfumes are stronger than colognes. Colognes have a more subtle smell and are not as strongly scented as perfumes.

Alcohol Base for Perfume

    4¼ teaspoons vodka
    1½ teaspoons distilled water
    60 drops of your essential oil blend

Mix the vodka and water and add your essential oils.

Alcohol Base for Cologne

    4½ teaspoons vodka
    2 teaspoons distilled water
    30 drops of your essential oil blend

Mix vodka and water before adding essential oils.

Carrier Oil Base for Perfume

    15-25 drops of essential oil blend
    1 tablespoon of jojoba oil

Perfumes made with a carrier oil blend are typically much stronger. It is important you never get in the mindset that using more essential oils is better. The oils are very strong and can damage your skin.

Choosing Your Oil Blends

While there are no set rules about blending scents, there are some tips you may want to follow in the beginning. You can certainly do as you wish, but some scents will not complement each other, and you will end up with a final product that is rather offensive. Here is a basic blending guide:

Spicy oils - Blend with citrus, oriental, and florals

Woodsy oil - Mix great with everything (excellent base notes)

Floral oils - Complemented by spicy, citrus, or woodsy scents

Mint oils - Blend well with earthy, woodsy, herb, and citrus oils

Now that you know what groups of oils blend well together, you need to know what oils fall into those groups. The following list is an idea of some of the more popular oils used to create beautiful perfumes and colognes. You can certainly experiment with some other lesser-known oils to create a unique scent.

Floral - Jasmine, rose, neroli, lavender

Earthy - Patchouli, vetiver, oakmoss

Spicy - Cinnamon, clove, nutmeg

Woodsy - Sandalwood, pine, cedarwood

Citrus - Orange, lime, lemon, bergamot

Minty - Peppermint, spearmint

Oriental - Nutmeg, patchouli

Herb - Rosemary, basil, marjoram

Have fun and try mixing and matching various scents until you come up with the right one for you and your mood. Each essential oil will give you a little extra pep in your step. When you are experimenting, start with small batches so if you don't like a particular scent, you won't end up wasting a lot of money and oils.

Chapter 8 - Hair Care

It isn't unheard of for people to spend hundreds of dollars every year taking care of their hair. Every one of us likes and needs something a little different to get that healthy mane we all desire. Some of us have skin conditions that leave our scalps dry and itchy while others have oily skin which tends to make our hair oily. Medicated shampoos or shampoos and conditioners designed to treat these issues can be costly.

Cost isn't the only deterrent from store-brand hair products. There are also harmful chemicals in some products you may not even be aware of. You can avoid all of that by making your own hair products at home that will take care of any problem you have with achieving that beautiful hair you love. Essential oils can be added to your base shampoo to take care of all kinds of skin conditions that leave the hair less than spectacular.

Top 10 Oils for Hair Care

- Tea tree
- Rosemary
- Lavender
- Sandalwood
- Chamomile

- Lemon
- Lemongrass
- Cypress
- Peppermint
- Clary sage

Dry Shampoo

1 tablespoon purified talc
4 drops tea tree oil
4 drops rosemary oil
4 drops lavender oil

Use a blender to mix ingredients. It is best to put talc in first and add a drop of oil at a time with the mixer on low speed. Store in a container with a lid. On days when you will not be using a wet shampoo, comb 1 to 2 teaspoons of the talc into your hair.

Hair Moisturizer

8 drops cedarwood oil
8 drops lavender oil
12 drops rosemary oil
1 ounce jojoba oil

Mix all ingredients in a plastic bottle. To use: add 1 teaspoon of the mixture to the hair. Massage oil into scalp and wrap head with a towel. Allow it to sit for 15 minutes. Wash your hair twice with shampoo to get rid of the oil. You can do this once a week or once a month depending on your needs.

Deep Hair Conditioner

2 teaspoons jojoba oil
6 drops sandalwood oil
3 drops chamomile oil
1 drop ylang-ylang oil

Put the oils in a small glass. Place the glass of oils into a bowl of very hot water. Allow the oil in the glass to get warm. Pour the oil on your hair, put your hair on top of your head, and wrap plastic wrap around your hair or use a shower cap. Wrap a towel around your head and allow the oil treatment to stay on your hair for 20 minutes. Wash your hair as you normally would after the 20 minutes is up.

Hair Loss

15 drops jojoba oil
8 drops carrot oil
7 drops rosemary oil
7 drops lavender oil
2 drops tea tree oil

Add the essential oils to 3 ounces of your regular shampoo. Do not add extra oils as this will not provide any benefit. Shampoo as you normally would. This will help reduce the amount of hair lost.

Hair Loss Massage

1½ ounces of rose water
1½ ounces distilled water
3 teaspoons apple cider vinegar
5 drops rosemary oil
6 drops jojoba oil
3 drops carrot oil

3 drops geranium oil

Mix all ingredients in a bottle. Store in the refrigerator. Add two teaspoons to the hair and gently massage into the scalp each morning. Shake well before each use.

Hair Loss Conditioner

2 ml jojoba oil (approx. ½ teaspoon)
8 drops evening primrose oil
2 drops geranium oil
2 drops palmarosa oil

Mix well and store in a sealed container. Apply conditioner once a week and allow it to sit on hair for 30 minutes. Use shampoo to rinse conditioner out of the hair.

Nightly Hair Loss Oil Treatment

3 drops rosemary oil
4 drops geranium oil
4 drops lavender oil
1 drop frankincense oil
4 drops cypress oil
2 drops cinnamon oil
2 drops juniper oil

Mix oils together and store in a container with a lid. Massage **only 1 drop** of oil mixture into the scalp every night before bed.

Oily Hair Treatment

9 drops ylang-ylang
9 drops lime oil
8 drops rosemary oil

2 tablespoons grapeseed oil

Mix all ingredients together. Apply 1 teaspoon to hair at night before bed. Use this treatment 3 times a week to control oily hair.

Hair Conditioner

1 tablespoon jojoba oil
1-3 drops rosemary oil

Mix ingredients and store in a small dish. You can double or triple this recipe for more frequent conditioning. To use: Wash hair as you normally would. Apply conditioner and allow to stay on hair for 15 minutes. Wash oil out of hair. You can use this treatment once a week or more often as needed.

Shampoo for Normal Hair

7 ounces unscented shampoo base
1 tablespoon jojoba
40 drops lavender oil
10 drops rosemary oil
5 drops ylang-ylang oil

Mix ingredients in a bottle. Use as you would a normal shampoo.

Shampoo to Treat Dandruff

½ cup liquid Castile soap
¼ cup canned coconut milk
¼ cup honey
2 tbsp fractionated coconut oil
1 tbsp vitamin E oil

10 drops lavender oil
10 drops tea tree oil
10 drops lemon oil
10 drops rosemary oil

Mix Castile soap, coconut milk, honey, vitamin E and coconut oil in plastic container. Add essential oils and shake well. Shake before each use. Use this shampoo as you would a store bought shampoo.

Herbal Shampoo

1 cup distilled water
¼ cup Castile soap
3 teaspoons dried rosemary
1 teaspoon lemongrass oil
2 teaspoons tea tree oil
½ teaspoon grapeseed oil

Boil the distilled water and add rosemary and lemongrass. Let the mixture steep for 30 minutes. Strain the water into a jar. Add the Castile soap, tea tree and grapeseed oil. Add a lid to the jar and shake well to get the oils and water to mix. Use as you would a store bought shampoo.

Shampoo for Fragile Hair

½ cup liquid Castile soap
¼ cup canned coconut milk
¼ cup honey
2 tbsp fractionated coconut oil
1 tbsp vitamin E oil
20 drops clary sage oil
15 drops lavender oil

15 drops orange oil

Mix Castile soap, coconut milk, honey, vitamin E and coconut oil in plastic container. Add essential oils and shake well. Shake before each use. Use this shampoo as you would a store bought shampoo.

Shampoo for Oily Scalp

½ cup Castile soap
½ cup distilled water
16 drops rosemary oil
2 drops peppermint oil

Add the Castile soap to a plastic container. Add your essential oils and mix. Add the water and shake again. Use as you would a store bought shampoo.

Shiny Hair Shampoo

1 cup distilled water
¼ cup Castile soap
2 teaspoons dried rosemary
2 teaspoons sweet almond oil
¼ teaspoon lemon oil

Boil the water and add rosemary. Allow mixture to steep for about 30 minutes. Strain the mixture and pour into a jar. Add almond and lemon oil and Castile soap. Shake well. This is a great recipe to give dull hair a bit of a shine.

Shampoo for Hair Growth

4 ounces of jojoba oil
12 drops rosemary oil
4 drops lavender oil
4 drops clary sage oil

4 drops thyme oil

Mix ingredients in a bottle. Shake well. Dampen your hair with warm water. Apply about a teaspoon of the oil mixture and rub it into the scalp and hair. Allow the oil to sit in your hair for 30 minutes. Wash thoroughly and allow your hair to air dry.

Chapter 9 - Personal Care

Personal hygiene is something we are all very fond of. We appreciate when we smell good and really appreciate it when others take the time to freshen up before heading to work or school. Feeling fresh and clean makes you feel good and many people will go to great lengths taking care of themselves and spend a lot of money doing so.

Sadly, there are plenty of personal care products that contain harsh chemicals that cause rashes and uncomfortable skin irritations. Some of the chemicals used to make us feel fresh and clean are actually known carcinogens. Carcinogens are the nasty chemicals that cause cancer. Fortunately, you can still smell good and feel clean without all of that when you opt to make your own personal care products with the addition of essential oils. You will also be saving a great deal of money by making your own products at home.

Top 10 Oils for Personal Care Products

- Peppermint
- Thyme
- Eucalyptus
- Lavender
- Tea tree

- Rosemary
- Bergamot
- Orange
- Spearmint
- Chamomile

Toothpaste - 1

    1 teaspoon of baking soda
    1 drop of peppermint oil

Mix the oil into the soda. The texture will still be a loose powder. It is a good idea to make a large batch of this and store it in a container with a lid.

Toothpaste - 2

    3 tablespoons baking soda
    2 tablespoons coconut oil
    5 drops peppermint oil
    5 drops spearmint oil

Mix well and use daily for teeth cleaning. This is safe for children. However, it is important they don't swallow the toothpaste. Baking soda is a natural tooth whitening agent and the peppermint and spearmint are natural bacteria fighters leaving your mouth clean and your teeth white.

Gingivitis Rinse

    3 drops thyme oil
    2 drops eucalyptus oil
    3 drops chamomile oil
    3 drops peppermint oil

1 teaspoon of brandy

Mix oils into brandy. Rinse mouth with the mixture and spit out.

Deodorant - 1

3 tablespoons baking soda
3 tablespoons shea butter
2 tablespoons cocoa butter
2 tablespoons corn starch
2 vitamin E gel caps
3 drops of orange essential oil

Mix all ingredients except for the essential oil. It is best to use a small jar to hold your deodorant. Add the oil and mix again. The deodorant will be an off-white color when applied and eventually fade to clear. Please note, this is a deodorant and not an antiperspirant. You will still sweat, but it won't stink!

Deodorant - 2 (Stick)

½ cup baking soda
¼ cup arrowroot
2 tablespoons of coconut oil
10 to 20 drops of either peppermint, lemon, or lavender oil

Stir the arrowroot, baking soda, and essential oil together. Add in the coconut oil and stir well. Put the mixture into an old deodorant container and let it sit for a few hours to solidify. Keep your homemade deodorant in a fairly cool place.

Mouthwash - 1

2 cups of water

20 drops of essential oil (peppermint or spearmint are excellent choices)

Pour the water into a dark glass bottle. You can buy these at your local health food store or online. Add the essential oil and mix well by shaking vigorously with a cap on the bottle. To use, put a little of the mouthwash in your mouth and swish around for 30 seconds. Spit out the mouthwash and your mouth will feel fresh. Do not swallow the mouthwash.

Mouthwash - 2

½ cup of water
2 teaspoons of baking soda
2 drops peppermint oil
2 drops tea tree oil

Mix ingredients together in a Mason jar with a lid. The baking soda will settle so make sure you shake well before each use. Swish and spit for a natural teeth whitening and cleaning routine.

Bodywash - 1

$^2/_3$ cup liquid Castile soap
¼ cup raw, unfiltered honey
2 teaspoons of a carrier oil (jojoba, almond, grapeseed, or olive)
1 teaspoon vitamin E oil
50 drops of your favorite essential oil (lavender, grapefruit, rosemary, peppermint, sweet orange, and patchouli are some examples)

Mix your ingredients together and store bodywash in a squirt container (check the dollar store for plastic ketchup and/or mustard bottles).

Bodywash - 2

2 cups liquid Castile soap
1 cup coconut oil
1 cup sweet almond oil
15 drops lavender oil
15 drops ylang-ylang oil
20 drops bergamot

Melt the coconut oil and add all ingredients to a glass jar. You can tweak this recipe to be more gentle and soothing by adding 20 drops of lavender and omitting the other essential oils.

Bath Melts

3 tablespoons of shea butter
3 tablespoons cocoa butter
¼ teaspoon honey lavender stress reliever tea (Yogi brand)
1 teaspoon of dried lavender flowers
30 drops of lavender oil
Silicone mold in any shape

Melt the cocoa and shea butter together either on the stove or in a glass bowl in the microwave. Open one tea bag and add the ¼ teaspoon to your melted butter mixture. Add the dried lavender to the mixture. Mix well and pour into your silicone mold. Add 2 drops of lavender oil to each mold. Allow the melts to cool completely and transfer to a jar with a lid. For a relaxing bath, add 1 melt to a tub of warm water.

Bath Salts

    2 cups Epsom salt
    1 cup sea salt
    ½ cup baking soda
    6 drops bergamot oil
    6 drops sweet orange oil
    3 drops lavender oil

Mix all ingredients together and store in a dark-colored jar. At bath time, pour about a cup of the salt mixture into the water. You will feel your tension start to ease away. It is an excellent bath additive before bed. You can increase this recipe to make a larger batch. This recipe makes enough for approximately 3 baths.

Skin Repair Bath Salts

    3 cups Dead Sea salt
    ½ cup baking soda
    6 drops palmarosa oil
    4 drops rose oil
    4 drops rose geranium oil
    1 drop vetiver oil
    1 drop ylang-ylang oil

Mix the salt and soda together in a dark-colored jar. Add the essential oils to the mix and stir well. Let the salt mixture sit for 24 hours before using. Add a cup to the bath for a reduction in itching caused by eczema or psoriasis.

Soothing Lavender Bath Salts

    3 cups Dead Sea salt
    ¼ cup liquid Castile soap

1 tablespoon vegetable glycerin
1 teaspoon white sugar
12 drops lavender oil
2 drops rose geranium oil
1 drop clary sage oil
1 drop chamomile oil

In a glass bowl, stir all the ingredients together EXCEPT the sea salt. Pour the salt into the bowl and stir thoroughly making sure the salt is completely coated with the oil mix. Store the mixture in a dark-colored glass jar. Let the mix sit for 24 hours before using. Add one cup to a bath for a bubbly, soothing bath.

Muscle Relaxing Bath Salts

3 cups Epsom salt
½ cup baking soda
6 drops bergamot oil
6 drops lemongrass oil
2 drops eucalyptus oil
2 drops rosemary oil

Mix the salt and soda together. Add the essential oils and stir well. Store in a dark-colored glass jar. Use one cup of salts per bath. This recipe can also be used to relieve congestion.

Lip Balm

1 tablespoon beeswax
2 tablespoons shea butter (cocoa butter can also be used)
2 tablespoons coconut oil
20 drops essential oil of your choice (peppermint, lavender, and wild orange are great options)

Melt the beeswax in a double boiler or put about an inch of water in a saucepan and jar filled with the beeswax in the pan. Add the shea butter and coconut oil and melt together. Once melted, turn off the heat but leave the jar in the hot water while adding the essential oil.

Use a glass dropper to fill about 18 empty lip balm tubes. Allow the mixture to completely cool and harden. This recipe will make a mildly firm Chapstick®. If you want it firmer, add a little more beeswax.

Shaving Cream

$^1/_3$ cup coconut oil

$^1/_3$ cup shea butter

2 tablespoons jojoba or sweet almond oil

2 tablespoons liquid Castile soap

2 drops cedarwood oil

2 drops lavender oil

1 drop lime oil

Make the shaving cream base by adding coconut oil and shea butter to a sauce pan. Warm over low heat until liquefied. Add jojoba or almond oil and mix well. Remove from heat and pour liquid mixture into a large bowl. Place bowl in the refrigerator until it hardens up. Once the mixture is hardened, use an egg beater to whip it. Add Castile soap and whip until the mixture is light and fluffy. Add the essential oils and whip the shaving cream another minute or so. Place your shaving cream in a jar with a lid and use every time you shave.

Aftershave - 1

¼ cup of water

20 drops of chamomile oil

Mix the water and oil. Use a cotton swab to rub over area. This is excellent for irritated skin.

Aftershave - 2

    ½ cup fresh aloe vera (can use gel if needed)

    1 tablespoon witch hazel

    ½ tablespoon water

    10 drops of oil (lavender, chamomile, rosemary, or orange)

Mix ingredients and store in a jar in the refrigerator. Use as needed.

Foot Powder

    1 tablespoon baking soda

    2 drops sage oil

    2 drops coriander oil

    2 drops spearmint oil

    2 ounces talc powder

Put talc inside a jar and add baking soda. Drop essential oils onto a cotton ball. Add the cotton ball to the jar and seal it. Shake ingredients and allow the powder to sit for 2 days. Use the powder on your feet or place inside shoes.

Sugar Scrub for Elbows and Heels

    $1^{1}/_{3}$ cups white sugar

    $^{2}/_{3}$ cup coconut oil

    20 drops lemon or peppermint oil

Melt coconut oil in microwave or on stove. Put oil in jar and add sugar and essential oil. Rub on heels and elbows to reduce rough skin.

Body Powder

10 drops peppermint oil
10 drops spruce oil
5 drops clove oil
5 drops spearmint oil
2 tablespoons corn starch

Mix ingredients together and apply powder as needed to feel fresh.

Insect Repellant

1½ ounces of distilled water
1½ ounces of high-proof alcohol
15 drops citronella oil
10 drops lavender oil
10 drops eucalyptus oil
5 drops lemongrass oil

Add water and alcohol to a clean spray bottle. Drop in essential oils and shake well to mix. Spray the skin with the mixture as needed to repel insects. You can omit the alcohol and use 3 ounces of water instead if you choose.

Conclusion

Thank you again for purchasing this book!

I hope the information contained herein was useful in helping you discover the many benefits associated with using essential oils. As you now know, essential oils provide us with an abundance of natural ways to enhance our lives and heal our ailments. There are literally hundreds of ways these oils can be used for the body and around the home. Thousands of years of humans successfully using these precious liquids has proven their worth.

I trust you are now ready to confidently begin using essentials oils following the numerous helpful recipes and instructions included in this handy reference. You'll, no doubt, benefit from incorporating essential oils in your daily life.

Also, don't forget to get my first book, **Essential Oils and Aromatherapy Basics: Your Ultimate Guide to Getting Started and Safely Using Essential Oils to Beat Stress, Cure Your Ailments, Boost Your Mood, and Provide Emotional Wellbeing**, if you need an indispensable primer to essential oils. It is packed with a wealth of useful information gathered from reliable and highly regarded sources. This comprehensive resource contains numerous helpful tips and guidance on buying, storing, and using essential oils so you can get started on the right path and with confidence.

Finally, if you enjoyed this book, please take the time to share your thoughts and post a review on Amazon. I would greatly appreciate it!

PS: You didn't forget to get your **FREE GIFT**, did you? Here's the link again just in case:

https://tinyurl.com/yy5rhpp3

Index

A

B

D

E

F

G

H

I

L

M

N

O

P

R

S

T

U

V

W

References

http://livesimply.me/index.php/2013/09/18/simple-homemade-moisturizer/

http://thecoconutmama.com/2013/10/50-uses-for-essential-oils/

http://www.diynatural.com/homemade-sunscreen/

http://altmedicine.about.com/od/massagethera2/ht/essential muscle.htm

http://www.experience-essential-oils.com/natural-muscle-relaxer.html

http://spiritualityhealth.com/articles/aromatherapy-cold-and-flu-season

http://www.mynaturalfamily.com/symptoms/eczema/essential-oils-for-eczema-treatment-ideas/

http://altmedicine.about.com/od/teatreeoil/a/teatreeoilacne.htm

https://blog.youngliving.com/sunburn-relief-with-essential-oils/#.U3tIYnZpyMQ

http://www.wisegeek.com/how-effective-is-lavender-oil-for-acne.htm

http://www.just4usoaps.com/athletes_foot.html#.U3tO43ZpyMQ

http://beautyeditor.ca/2011/08/23/ever-made-your-own-face-mask-whip-up-these-budget-friendly-beauty-treatments-to-get-glowing-the-natural-way-no-birkenstocks-required/

http://www.easy-aromatherapy-recipes.com/homemade-face-masks.html

http://www.aromaweb.com/recipes/massageoil.asp

http://birchhillhappenings.com/recipes/massage.htm

http://essentialoilbenefits.org/top-10-essential-oils-sleep-insomnia/

REFERENCES

http://www.biosourcenaturals.com/essential-oils-for-arthritis.htm

http://www.naturalcosmeticnews.com/focus/make-your-own-natural-personal-care-products-with-5-easy-recipes/

http://www.essentialoilbusinessdoterra.com/natural-homemade-deodorant-recipes-with-essential-oils.html

http://www.easy-aromatherapy-recipes.com/aromatherapy-for-depression.html#.U33sQ3ZpyMQ

http://www.doterraeveryday.com/diy-mouthwash-recipe-made-with-essential-oils-for-a-fresh-clean-mouth/

http://birchhillhappenings.com/motion.htm

http://www.sunwarrior.com/news/make-your-own-winter-mood-enhancing-essential-oil-blend/

http://www.diynatural.com/homemade-natural-mouthwash/

http://www.diynatural.com/homemade-body-wash/

http://marycrimmins.com/diy-chemical-free-moisturizing-body-wash/

http://happymoneysaver.com/homemade-relaxing-bath-melts/

http://www.natural-homeremedies-for-life.com/homemade-aftershave.html

http://www.mommypotamus.com/mamas-homemade-soothing-burn-salve/

http://wellnessmama.com/7055/homemade-lip-chap-recipe/

http://www.thankyourbody.com/natural-body-spray-recipe/

http://www.mommypotamus.com/sandalwood-and-vanilla-solid-perfume-recipe/

http://www.aromaweb.com/recipes/depression.asp

http://www.aromaweb.com/recipes/sstress.asp

http://www.easy-aromatherapy-recipes.com/bath-salt-recipe.html

http://www.easy-aromatherapy-recipes.com/lavender-bubble-bath-salts.html

http://www.easy-aromatherapy-recipes.com/salt-bath-recipe.html

http://www.experience-essential-oils.com/home-remedies-for-anxiety.html

http://www.theprairiehomestead.com/2014/03/essential-oil-diffuser-blends.html#sthash.EmA1wWyy.dpbs

http://bodysoulmind.net/body/essential-oils-and-aromatherapy-to-heal-bladder-infections-and-cystitis

http://www.family-essential-oils.com/basic-first-aid-instructions.html

http://ournourishingroots.com/how-to-treat-hives-naturally/

http://www.homemademommy.net/2014/01/natural-home-remedies-for-ear-infections.html

http://theelliotthomestead.com/2013/12/trying-to-get-rid-of-your-eczema-try-this/

http://www.aromaweb.com/articles/aromatherapy-essential-oils-for-headaches.asp

http://www.easy-aromatherapy-recipes.com/therapeutic-massage-oil.html

http://www.essentialoils.co.za/treatment/heartburn.htm

http://www.onlynature.co.uk/menopause.html

http://www.aromaweb.com/recipes/memory.asp

http://www.essentialoils.co.za/treatment/sore-throat.htm

http://www.greenlivingladies.com/2014/01/addadhd-and-improving-focus-and.html

http://gianelloni.wordpress.com/2014/02/03/young-living-essential-oil-testimonies-part-3-autism-adhd-asthma-allergies-eczema/

http://birchhillhappenings.com/warts.htm

REFERENCES

http://thecrunchymoose.com/2014/03/varicose-vein-attacking-body-butter.html

http://everydayroots.com/clove-toothache-remedy

http://birchhillhappenings.com/mouth.htm

http://essentialoilblogging.com/2013/05/25/natural-remedies-for-poison-ivy-oak-and-sumac-using-essential-oils/

http://www.dreamingearth.com/blog/essential-oils-for-poison-ivy/

http://www.essentialoils.co.za/hair-care.htm

http://birchhillhappenings.com/recipes/hairskin.htm

http://www.aromaweb.com/recipes/default.asp?PHPSESSID=36cf377e9912353739050ea9cab46ee8

http://www.essentialoils.co.za/recipes.htm

http://doterrablog.com/diy-essential-cologne/

http://www.easy-aromatherapy-recipes.com/essential-oils-perfume.html

http://www.commonsensehome.com/make-perfume/

http://shalommama.com/homemade-shampoo

http://www.homemademommy.net/2014/02/homemade-rosemary-peppermint-shampoo.html

http://mypurepursuit.blogspot.com/p/shampoo-recipes_19.html

http://www.essentialoils.co.za/treatment/abdominal-pain.htm

http://www.naturesgift.com/firstaid_howto.htm

http://herbs.lovetoknow.com/Eucalyptus_Oil_Fibromyalgia

http://blog.naturalhealthyconcepts.com/2013/06/05/aromatherapy-benefits-essential-oil-recipes/

http://www.theherbsplace.com/Essential_Oil_Recipes_For_Specific_Health_Issues_sp_178.html

http://www.exhibithealth.com/general-health/7-natural-remedies-for-shingles-750/

http://wellnessmama.com/3527/natural-vapor-rub/

http://www.dreamingearth.com/catalog/pc/Aromatherapy-Recipes-d3.htm

http://www.aromaticsinternational.com/index.php?route=product/recipe

http://www.natural-aromatherapy-benefits.com/thievesoilrecipe.html

http://veggieconverter.com/diy-presents-coconut-oil-sugar-scrub/

http://dontmesswithmama.com/6-personal-care-products-for-men/

http://www.easy-aromatherapy-recipes.com/natural-hair-remedies.html

http://www.livestrong.com/article/213767-how-to-mix-essential-oils-for-hair-growth/

Report dead links here:

softpresspub@gmail.com

Made in United States
Orlando, FL
10 July 2024

48805808R00054